CAREERS IN

RECREATIONAL THERAPY

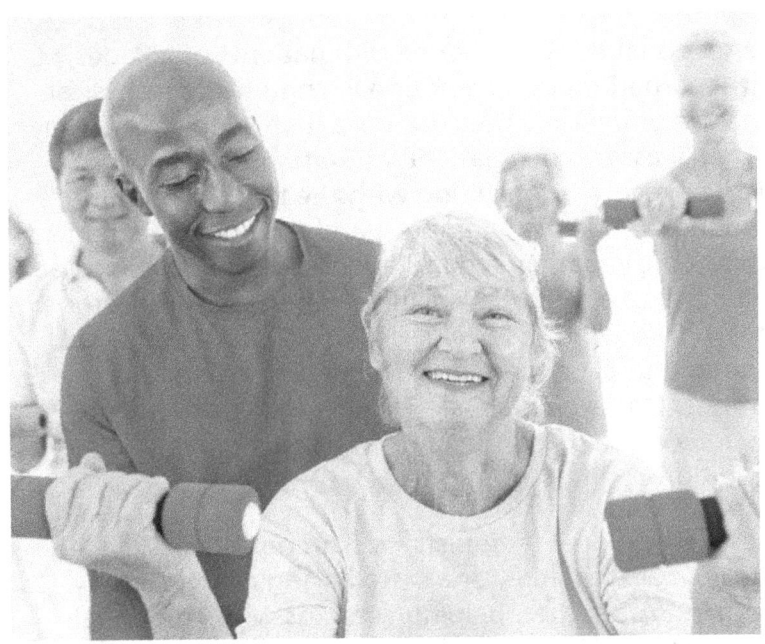

RECREATIONAL THERAPY IS ONE OF the most popular fields in the healthcare industry. It is not surprising considering recreational therapists are paid to have fun with their patients. Recreational therapy is exactly what it sounds like – using recreation and leisure activities as a therapeutic device. For example, horseback riding can offer numerous benefits to a teenager with Cerebral Palsy. It can improve physical functionality and neurological connections, provide opportunities for social inclusion, and overcome depression through freedom of movement. Adaptive swimming, one of the most common forms of recreational therapy, is a safe, low-impact way to regain strength after a heart attack, develop motor skills in children with disabilities, or treat the cognitive and emotional effects of Autism. The possibilities are endless, but the overall concept is that recreational activities can better a person's quality of life.

Recreational therapists work with patients of all ages, with a broad range of emotional, cognitive, or physical illnesses or injuries. They do more than simply play. They carefully assess each patient's situation by reviewing medical records, consulting with the medical team, meeting with family members, and talking to the patient. Based on the patient's goals and interests, the therapist will develop a treatment plan designed specifically for that individual. It may involve any kind of activity – art, drama, music, dance, sports, games, or community outings. Once the plan is in place, regular treatment sessions begin using fun stuff to help improve their condition.

Most recreational therapists work in hospitals, skilled nursing care facilities, or assisted living centers. Many work in VA facilities, helping veterans with emotional issues like PTSD or physical disabilities like amputations. Recreational therapy is extremely popular in nursing homes where the elderly need help keeping up their fine motor skills, brain function, and mental well-being. Recreational therapists can also be found working in school systems, prisons, halfway houses, special education departments, parks and recreation departments, and outpatient centers for substance abuse or rehabilitation.

A bachelor's degree is required to become a certified recreational therapist. If you are not ready to spend four years in college, there is an alternative. It only takes two years to earn an associate degree, which is the minimum requirement for an entry-level position. However, an associate degree does not qualify you for certification, and without certification opportunities for pay raises and advancement are limited. A certified recreational therapist earns an average yearly income of roughly $50,000. Without a bachelor's degree and certification, the best you can expect is around $30,000.

It is also possible to enter the field as a recreational therapy aide with no more than a high school diploma. This is a good way to experience what the work is really like before committing to the necessary training.

Recreational therapy is a career that is both enjoyable and challenging. You will be paid to have fun while helping people achieve a better quality of life. It offers variety and flexibility – your training will prepare you to work with any population and build on your interests. If you are looking for a career in the healthcare field where patients will be happy to see you, read on.

WHAT YOU CAN DO NOW

MAKE HIGH SCHOOL COUNT. BECOMING a recreational therapist requires a bachelor's degree. Make a list of the colleges you are interested in and check their admission requirements to make sure you are taking all the necessary classes. Science classes should be a priority, particularly biology, anatomy, and psychology. Take AP courses if they are available. Any classes in fitness and wellness will be helpful. Keep your grades up. Admission officers want to see a GPA of at least 3.0.

Get involved in activities that interest you. Common activities that recreational therapists specialize in include: arts and crafts, dance, music, drama, writing, sports, board games, and puzzles. You can pursue these through classes, clubs, or summer camps.

Explore the field. Talk to professional recreational therapists about the work they do. Ask your school counselor to help you arrange job shadowing. Spending a day with a therapist at work is an excellent way to learn what this career is really like on a daily basis. Be prepared with plenty of questions and ask for advice.

To get an even better sense of what this career entails, volunteer at a hospital, rehabilitation center, or home for the elderly. In addition to providing invaluable experience, it will add weight to your college application.

There are a number of professional associations for recreational therapists. With the exception of the American Therapeutic Recreation Association, most are dedicated to a particular specialization such as music, dance, or art. Visit a variety of association websites to learn more about the particular types of recreational therapy you can get involved in.

HISTORY OF THE CAREER

THE BENEFITS OF SOME RECREATION experiences have been recognized for thousands of years, but recreation as an organized and professionally designed form of therapy did not emerge until the 19th century. One person is credited with bringing recreational therapy into the healthcare setting. That person was renowned British nurse, Florence Nightingale.

It was during the Crimean War that Nightingale was tasked with reforming the profession of nursing. Her efforts went much farther and included changing the way patients were routinely treated. When she arrived in a British military hospital in Eastern Europe in 1854, she was appalled to find that following surgery patients were parked on cots in dark and colorless rooms, left alone to live or die. Nightingale asserted that patient outcomes would improve in a more stimulating environment. She wrote to healthcare administrators, describing how recovery would be faster and more certain when patients did needlework, cared for pets, listened to music, and wrote stories. Without waiting for permission, she arranged singing classes and had friends send costumes for a theatrical group that patients organized. As the hospitals continued to fill up, she was dubbed the Mother of Hospital Recreation.

Recreational therapy was slow to be adopted in the US healthcare environment. The first major step forward came in 1889 with the founding of Hull House in Chicago. It started as a community center that provided recreation and other services to the poor. It later offered classes for hospital workers who cared for the insane. The courses demonstrated how to use games, arts, crafts, and various hobby activities to "reach" mentally ill patients.

In 1903, the New York School of Philanthropy started offering a one-year course in social work. In addition to the usual topics of housing and education, it included the study of Nightingale's thesis that certain recreation experiences could be utilized to improve health.

Recreational therapy was first defined as a new type of psychotherapy in 1909. The Journal of the Indiana State Medical Association reported that, when applied correctly, recreational therapy could have a positive impact in the management of functional neuroses. The Journal was careful to point out that it was not enough to instruct a patient to take a walk or go to the theater. In order to see a positive response, it was necessary to ascertain what the particular patient enjoyed.

The principles of recreational therapy were fully recognized and established during World War I. The American Red Cross spent an unprecedented amount of money building 52 recreation centers at military hospitals. Called convalescent houses, the centers were completed shortly before the end of the war in 1918. The Red Cross hired teachers from Columbia University to train and supervise several hundred "highly specialized and technically trained recreation and entertainment personnel." They also hired an army of recreation consultants to visit and teach hospital staff how to use play to encourage disabled patients to push the limits of physical possibilities. Recommended activities included music, dance, gardening, day trips, drama, games, and social recreation. The training service was titled Hospital Recreation Work.

At the end of the war, a two-year experiment began to explore the effectiveness of recreational therapy in the Illinois state mental health system. The program included games, dancing, marching, and gymnastics designed to meet the level of individual patients' cognitive ability. According to a report on the project, the results were clearly positive. A leading psychiatrist involved with the experiment, speaking to the managing officers of state institutions, said recreation could provide more effective treatment than medicine, physiotherapy, or occupational therapy.

During World War II, the Red Cross again recruited a large number of hospital recreation workers. Most recruits were college-educated women who were trained in recreation leadership and how to work with military patients. These workers were needed in a hurry and the training program was distilled to a total of seven weeks. By 1945, the number of hospital recreation workers topped 1,800. The war years provided a huge body of new knowledge gained through experience working with thousands of patients. Many new techniques emerged and workers learned to adapt equipment and activities for patients with various disabilities. It was also the first time that many doctors and psychologists saw recreational therapy being effectively applied in the treatment process.

As doctors returned from the war, word spread and the demand for recreational therapy programs grew across the country. The VA established a recreational therapy program in 1952 that was designed to help doctors improve patient recovery. A year later, the profession got a big boost when the National Association of Recreational Therapists (NART) was established. Soon after came the Council for the Advancement of Hospital Recreation. The Council's purpose was to establish qualifying standards for hospital recreation personnel. It also established the national registration program that later morphed into today's certification program.

Throughout the 1950s and 60s, physicians extolled the virtues of recreational therapy at meetings and seminars throughout the country. There were differing schools of thought. Some believed that recreation could only be used to elevate the quality of living rather than correcting a disorder. Others believed it was potentially much more powerful than that. Some physicians in the latter camp conducted research to test their hypotheses. For example, in one of the first scientific studies in the field, cardiologist Joseph B. Wolffe experimented with two groups of patients in separate cardiac units. One group received focused recreation activities daily while patients in the second unit received none. Among the findings, Wolffe reported that those in the treatment group made far fewer requests for sleep medications than those in the second group. Wolffe was clearly impressed by the recreational therapists involved in his study. He said, "They are professionals, skilled in the arts of recreational therapy, capable of making clinical observations that are on a par with those produced by the best of physicians." He concluded that a recreational therapist could be an invaluable member of the medical team that includes the cardiologist, neuropsychiatrist, surgeon, and other specialists.

WHERE YOU WILL WORK

THERE ARE ABOUT CLOSE TO 19,000 recreational therapists at work in the US. They work in a variety of settings ranging from parks and recreations departments, to substance abuse centers, to hospice care facilities.

Hospitals employ the largest number of recreational therapists. In fact, more than 35 percent of all recreational therapists work in hospitals, both public and private. Recreational therapy is a mainstay in many government facilities. State hospitals, particularly mental health facilities, always have recreational therapists on staff. At the federal level, the armed forces and especially the VA operate hospitals that provide therapy for service personnel. Private hospitals and HMOs are also among those facilities that usually employ recreational therapists.

Nursing care facilities and assisted living centers account for another 20 percent of recreational therapist jobs. In this environment, the clientele is primarily the elderly. There are other residential (inpatient) care facilities with recreational therapists on staff. These facilities tend to specialize in treating specific problems such as substance abuse, eating disorders, and other types of mental health issues.

Local and state governments hire another 20 percent of all recreational therapists. These are in addition to hospitals. They work in parks and recreation departments, community centers, school systems, special education departments, and outpatient centers for substance abuse or rehabilitation.

Work Environment

Most recreational therapists do their planning, patient assessment, and other administrative work in offices. However, this could not be described as a desk job. These professionals spend most of their time working with patients in various locations. This may be in a clinical setting or out in the community. For example, a therapist may travel between schools helping art teachers with struggling students. Even therapists stationed in hospitals can get out and about. They often take their patients to parks, sports fields, or swimming pools for therapeutic activities.

Most recreational therapists work full time, but about one in four works part time. Evening and weekend scheduling is common, especially for those employed by outpatient facilities.

THE WORK YOU WILL DO

RECREATIONAL THERAPISTS, ALSO referred to as therapeutic recreation specialists, provide treatment services and recreation activities for individuals with disabilities or illnesses. Millions of people of all ages live with a chronic illness, mental health issue, cognitive impairment, or physical disability. Sometimes the issue is temporary, such as an accident victim going through rehabilitation or a person recovering from a stroke. In other cases, the condition is permanent, such as a child born with cerebral palsy or a young adult with MS. For many of these people, even the simplest activities that most of us enjoy may be quite difficult, if not impossible. Yet, there are ways to help improve functioning and the quality of life on every level. This is the goal of the recreational therapist, the trained professional who uses fun activities as a therapeutic treatment.

Using a variety of techniques, from horseback riding to acting in plays, recreational therapists improve and maintain the physical, mental, and emotional well-being of their patients. They help individuals reduce depression, overcome stress and anxiety, recover basic motor skills, improve reasoning abilities, regain balance, build confidence, and form social relationships. Utilizing leisure activities is a proven way to help patients participate more fully in life, enjoy greater independence, and reduce or eliminate the effects of their illness or disability.

Recreational therapists are valued members of the professional team that may include doctors, surgeons, nursing staff, psychologists and/or psychiatrists, physical therapists, speech therapists, social workers, and teachers. Their work often mirrors that of the occupational therapist. The goals may be very similar – both seek to enable patients with disabilities to lead better lives, but the modalities are quite different. Occupational therapy often focuses on a narrow goal, such as strengthening a limb or practicing a necessary task in order to be more productive. Recreational therapy's purpose has a wider scope, to improve overall quality of life for patients who have physical or cognitive challenges. It is meant to help a patient experience enjoyment of life and feel a part of the community.

Every recreational therapy plan is unique to the patient, taking into consideration the patient's individual interests and overall goals. For a physically disabled person, for example, that could mean something as simple as finding a group activity that will foster new friendships to playing adaptive sports such as wheelchair basketball with the goal of someday participating in the Paralympics.

What Do They Do?

The recreational therapist must develop a treatment plan that meets the needs of the individual patient. No two patients are alike – they all have their own problems to address, as well as personal interests. A treatment plan starts with an assessment. This phase begins with preliminary research, which might include reviewing medical records, test results, mental health evaluations, and firsthand observations of medical staff and other human services workers. There may be a meeting with family members to gain insight into the patient's background, personality, preferences, and interests.

Once this research is completed, the therapist meets with the new patient. Therapists ask patients their opinion on where they are in their care, what their abilities and disabilities are, and what their personal goals might be. Then comes the basic question: What do you enjoy doing? The answers to these questions will be used to create a treatment plan unique to each individual client.

Treatment plans revolve around intervention modalities such as creative arts (painting, crafts, music, dance, and drama, for example), sports, relaxation techniques, gardening, games, group outings, animal therapy, and field trips. The prescribed treatment activities take place on a regular basis, such as daily or weekly. One of the main responsibilities of the recreational therapist is to counsel and encourage patients to participate in the activities and acquire new skills. During treatment sessions, recreational therapists observe, analyze, and record patients' participation and responses. Progress is carefully tracked and treatment is modified as needed.

Specializations

A trained recreational therapist is capable of working with any population, but most therapists specialize in treating specific types of patients. Their specialties are usually based on personal interests. Once they have worked in that area for a while, they may pursue certification for their specialty.

One of the most common specialties is geriatrics. This is a good specialty to get into because it is the area with the greatest need. One of the biggest issues with the elderly is isolation and loneliness, which can lead to depression and even failing health. The therapist would counter these problems by concentrating on increasing social interaction. Activities would be planned for groups rather than individuals, whether it is exercising, walking, dancing, swimming, or playing games. Activities outside the nursing home or assisted living center are especially important. A group picnic in the park is a perfect example of a healthy outing.

Another popular specialty is pediatrics, which may include working with infants, toddlers, children, adolescents, and young adults. Patients may be ill, such as children with cancer. Others may have cognitive or physical disabilities. The goal of the pediatric recreational therapist is to identify and improve functional abilities and reduce the effects of illness or disability on children through leisure and play. Individual and group activities can take place at bedside, in clinic areas, on school grounds, in teen centers, or outside.

Pediatric recreational therapists can be especially helpful in the hospital environment. They can improve the hospital experience – which can be downright scary for any child. They help children understand what is happening to them through age-appropriate expressive play. Playful activities can also provide distraction and support during difficult physical therapy sessions and medical procedures. Some recreational therapists work with terminally ill children, using animal visits, favorite games, music, and plays to boost their spirits.

Rehabilitation is another major area of specialization. Leisure activities can help rebuild physical strength and functionality. For example, a right-handed stroke patient may suffer some level of paralysis on the right side of the body. The therapist would choose activities that promote improved coordination on the left side, such as swinging a golf club, casting a fishing rod, tossing a beanbag, or shooting baskets with the left arm. For patients recovering from major surgery, the goal would be promoting muscle strength, stability, and flexibility through activities such as aquatic therapy or light aerobic dance.

Recreational Therapy Aide/Assistant

A recreational therapy aide, sometimes known as a recreational therapy assistant, is a person who provides support to the certified recreational therapist. That support is usually related to the therapy itself. Aides never do assessments, but they may do background research, help come up with plans, gather supplies, assist with scheduling, and coordinate group activities. They may also be asked to monitor the success of an activity and report any signs of progress or setbacks to the supervising therapist.

The main focus of the aide is on facilitating activities and helping patients participate. What this might entail depends mostly on the situation. For example, an assisted living home might want the recreational therapy aide to cook breakfast, lead a field trip to a shopping center, or provide transportation to medical or religious services. The goal is to help residents stay active and mentally alert. The work of an aide employed by a juvenile detention center will conduct all services on-site. That might include leading social games such as trivia or organizing other group activities aimed at encouraging positive social interactions.

It is common for recreational therapists to begin their careers working as aides. It is a good way to determine if the field is of lasting interest before investing in the necessary education to become a certified recreational therapist. The time spent as a working aide helps satisfy certain experience requirements and often makes the needed coursework easier. It can also help you to land a job with prior work experience as an aide on your résumé.

PROFESSIONALS TALK ABOUT THEIR WORK

I Work With Elderly Women

"I work in a clinic associated with a teaching hospital. My patients are mostly older women who have been hospitalized. Sometimes I see them while they are still in the hospital, providing guided bedside exercise and teaching relaxation techniques. Once they are discharged there are a number of options. It is a large facility, and I have many resources at my disposal. There is a pool, a relaxation room, a gym, craft and play/game rooms, and a family center. I work with patients in my office, but only until I've developed a treatment plan for them. The relaxation room is a favorite, especially among new discharges. It is furnished with massage tables and vibroacoustic recliners that emit vibrations and soothing musical sounds. There is also a weekly pain clinic where my team works on reducing patients' discomfort.

Because this is a teaching hospital, part of my job is to speak about various aspects of my specialty. At the hospital, I talk to groups of rehabilitation professionals about the importance of leisure activities and also to oncology nurses about cancer-related fatigue. Outside the hospital, I talk to state parks and recreation associations about the role that recreation can play in recovery and continuing overall health.

I considered several kinds of therapy before training to become a recreational therapist. I chose this field because it deals with the whole person. These women are often referred to me to help them deal with recovery after surgery, but when I talk to them during the assessment, deeper issues often emerge. There may be memory problems, lack of confidence in decision-making, mood swings, depression, and isolation. Did you know that loneliness can impede healing and shorten your life? I take these issues into account along with their abilities and interests, to plan their treatment.

The best thing about this work is making people happy. Seeing a group of women smiling and laughing with their pool noodles makes my day. It is also very creative work. Treatment plans can't be cookie cutter. Each plan is uniquely individualized. I like that. Just as each person is different, each day is different. The word boredom isn't even in my vocabulary."

I Work With At-Risk Youth

"My original career goal was to become a nurse. While in college, I worked part time in a hospital as a phlebotomist (a healthcare specialist trained in drawing blood for testing or donation). Everyone who came to see me had a look of fear and dread on their face. I mentioned off-handedly to my counselor that I hated being seen as a 'vampire.' He suggested that I look up 'recreational therapist' in the school catalog. It stated that the prerequisites were very similar to nursing. My counselor pointed out that I already had completed two years of schooling, so if I switched my major it would only be two more years to become a recreational therapist. There was no apparent downside to changing course so I went for it.

One of the requirements for graduation was to complete an internship. My three-month internship was in a group home for abused and neglected children. The experience opened my eyes to an entirely different kind of work than I had anticipated. That's the beauty of this field. A recreational therapist can work with many different populations, and yet the work itself can be different within each group. I'm certified in pediatrics, but I can work with kids who have cancer, young children with cognitive disabilities, or at-risk kids who are struggling in school. It's good to know that if I ever decide I don't want to work with at-risk kids anymore, I still have many other options.

I have worked in several environments including halfway houses for boys who are transitioning between juvenile detention and returning home, and inner city group homes for troubled boys whose next stop would be prison if intervention failed. It's an awesome responsibility, but I find the work enjoyable and deeply rewarding. My job is to inject positive activities in the form of recreation into their lives. It is very individualized and I choose from a wide variety of activities. I might have former gang members making friendship bracelets (they resisted, but it turned out to be a favorite activity), teaming up for basketball tournaments, going horseback riding, cooking for a potluck meal, or caring for rescue pets. Many times, I find I am exposing them to things they have never experienced – or even heard of. Can you believe there are kids who have never heard of hockey?

I know I could make more money as a nurse, but this field is special. Every day I get to help kids take another step towards becoming a whole person with a positive outlook on life. Accomplishing this invites lateral thinking and creativity like no other career I've seen."

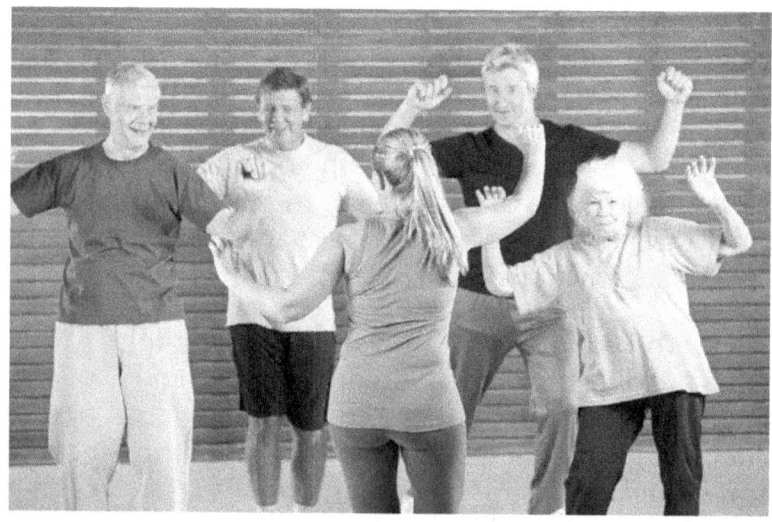

PERSONAL QUALIFICATIONS

WHILE PREPARING TO BECOME A recreational therapist, having an aptitude for science and a keen interest in how the mind works will certainly help you build a foundation of necessary knowledge. Once working in the field, there are a number of personal skills that will help you succeed in this career.

The number one motivation for recreational therapists is a strong desire to help others improve and enjoy their lives. It is not a career for the selfish or impatient. The best recreational therapists always put the needs of others first and are truly interested in their well-being. In return, they are rewarded with the deep satisfaction that comes from helping people with different emotional, physical, and mental challenges.

A high level of compassion is necessary. You must be comfortable working with people who are sick or disabled. Patients may be in pain or under emotional stress. They need to be treated with kindness, empathy, and respect. Patience is key. Some patients will require more time and special attention than others. They may get frustrated and angry about the slow pace of progress. A good recreational therapist acts as a cheerleader, gently urging them to continue towards their goals.

Good communications skills are essential. Being an active listener is especially important. In order to determine the best course of treatment, a recreational therapist must first listen carefully to each patient's problems and concerns. Recreational therapy is a fun job, but it is more than being a camp counselor or event planner. It often involves meaningful discussions of feelings and emotions.

It takes good speaking skills along with active listening skills to elicit honest responses from patients. Recreational therapists must also be able to give clear directions during activities and instructions on coping techniques to utilize at home.

Recreational therapists must possess mental, emotional, and physical strength. Working with injured and ill patients every day is not easy. Successful recreational therapists are able to handle highly emotional situations. It also helps to have a sense of humor.

In addition to being mentally and emotionally challenging, the work is physically taxing. You will be on your feet most of the day, and you will need to be able to provide physical assistance to patients with mobility issues.

Leadership skills are needed to engage and motivate patients to participate in therapeutic activities. Resourcefulness is a big plus when planning, developing, and implementing effective programs. Treatment plans are customized for each individual patient. You must be creative and flexible when adapting activities to meet each patient's needs. Because you will be planning activities for a variety of patients, you also need to be highly organized.

ATTRACTIVE FEATURES

THE VAST MAJORITY OF RECREATIONAL THERAPISTS report a high level of job satisfaction. There are a number of reasons for this, but the most common include the following.

The number one positive aspect is the opportunity to help others. It is also the main reason most recreational therapists choose this career. Roughly nine out of 10 say they feel the work they do makes other people's lives better. The progress made over time is especially satisfying because it is tangible. The level of pain is diminished, depression lifted, and mobility restored. It can be a joy to watch.

You get paid to do what you enjoy. What other job pays you to swim, dance, play board games, go on field trips, or put on costumes and create a play just for the fun of it? And, it can be fun for everybody. What other healthcare professional has patients lining up in front of the elevator eagerly waiting to see them?

There is considerable flexibility in this career. You can work full time, part time, or have multiple jobs. You can choose a static work setting such as a hospital, or move around among different locations like those who work in school systems.

There is also variety to this work. You have the option to work with any demographic from kids to the elderly. You can also choose any sort of patient population. You can work exclusively with veterans, recovering substance abusers, psychiatric patients, those with developmental disabilities, or people with certain chronic illnesses. Forget about becoming bored!

You can become certified in almost anything that interests you. Want to try cardio drumming? Story telling? Training kids for the Paralympics? Following what makes you happy is a great way to stay in love with your job.

Recreational therapy is an up-and-coming healthcare profession. There is great demand creating many jobs everywhere. You can live the small town life if you want, but the real action is in the cities. Wherever you go, you can count on finding a position with exceptional job security.

Recreational therapy is a fascinating study of the body/-mind connection. It offers the unique opportunity to come up with creative approaches to help individual patients improve their quality of life. Whatever makes a patient happy, also makes them healthy. While some settings provide more opportunities for creativity than others, all rely on the therapist's ability to discover what activity will elicit a positive response.

UNATTRACTIVE ASPECTS

MANY PEOPLE ARE ATTRACTED TO THIS CAREER. Although the demand is growing fast and there are plenty of jobs being created, there is often competition in certain areas. The best way to get an edge on the competition is to have more education and experience than other candidates. Of course, that takes more time and effort than some people want to invest.

The job is fun, but it is not suitable for everyone. Not everyone is a people person, and not everyone is comfortable delving into deep emotional waters to assess the needs of patients. You also need to be comfortable working with people who are sick, disabled, and suffering. Even people who get into the field with the best of intentions may discover they cannot deal with certain bodily functions.

The work can be physically demanding. Not all recreational therapy involves physical activity, but most jobs do. Therapists are usually on their feet most of the time. Depending on the type of patients being treated, recreational therapists may need the strength to lift patients or help them move their limbs.

Many patients are dealing with a high level of stress from physical and emotional pain. It can be difficult for a therapist to deal with, day after day. Not everyone is up to the emotional challenge. Therapy treatments can go on over a long period of time. To avoid succumbing to stress themselves, recreational therapists must learn to face every situation with a positive attitude. It is necessary for your own health and well-being.

The money is at the low end for healthcare careers. It is a livable wage, but nowhere near what closely related professionals like occupational and physical therapists make. On the other hand, the educational requirements are lower as well. Other types of therapists need a master's or doctoral degree, while a recreational therapist only needs an associate or bachelor's degree.

EDUCATION AND TRAINING

BECOMING A RECREATIONAL THERAPIST requires a college education. Most recreational therapists earn a bachelor's degree in recreation therapy, which qualifies them to become certified. It is also possible to choose a closely related field such as recreation and leisure studies. Undergraduate work takes four years to complete. In addition to general education requirements, courses in a recreational therapy program include:

Human anatomy and physiology

Medical and psychiatric terminology

The use of medical equipment and assistive devices

Client assessment

Characteristics of illnesses and disabilities

Medical technology

Physical and behavioral sciences

Recreational therapy administration

Abnormal psychology

There are typically elective courses in working with specific types of clients such as the elderly or the disabled.

Most recreational therapy programs also require a hands-on work component. This may be an internship or a volunteer position. Either will qualify if the student is working under the supervision of a certified recreational therapist.

Graduate Degrees

There are graduate degree programs for those who intend to advance into administrative roles in the field. Graduate degree programs can usually be completed within one to two years, depending on whether the student is part time or full time.

A Master of Science in Recreational Therapy degree curriculum is focused on more advanced forms of therapy as well as management and administration topics. Coursework typically covers subjects such as program planning and development, recreation and leisure research methods, recreational therapy finance management, and advanced assessment and evaluation of patient health. Graduate students can also concentrate their studies in a particular treatment area such as art therapy or aquatic therapy. A master's thesis or major project is generally required.

Associate Degree

There is also a way to enter the field with only two years of college. An associate degree program in recreational therapy only requires a high school diploma or GED for admission. This degree can open doors to a number of entry-level jobs including:

Recreational therapy aide/assistant

Rehabilitation activity director

Special recreation program leader

Adult activity coordinator

Assisted living program service coordinator

Coursework involves less general education and is more concerned with the practical aspects of recreational therapy. Typical classes include the core recreational therapy courses such as patient interaction counseling, and recreation for special needs. There is also a choice of relevant classes in music, art, drama, and social dance. In addition to classroom instruction, students are required to gain hands-on experience in the field.

Training

On-the-job training is a common requirement for newly hired recreational therapists. Employer training programs may be formal or informal, and the length will depend on the situation. For example, a children's hospital might have a six-week training program that teaches recreational therapists the most effective methods to communicate and interact with children and adolescents. On the other hand, a treatment center for people with developmental disabilities might provide a few hours of instruction related to preventing clients from posing a danger to themselves or others.

Licensing

Most states do not require recreational therapists to be licensed. The four exceptions are New Hampshire, North Carolina, Oklahoma, and Utah. Specific licensing requirements can be obtained from the state's medical board, but they are generally a combination of specific education and experience, a degree conferred by an accredited institution, internship experience, and a successful score on an examination. The other 46 states accept certifications as evidence that recreational therapists are qualified to practice.

Certification

Most employers, especially hospitals and other clinical facilities, prefer to hire certified recreational therapists. The Certified Therapeutic Recreation Specialist (CTRS) credential is offered by the National Council for Therapeutic Recreation Certification (NCTRC). The CTRS demonstrates to employers that the therapists have completed advanced studies, training, and substantial work experience. To be eligible for certification, candidates must have a bachelor's degree (or equivalent education), one to five years of experience working in the field (depending on the amount of education), and successful passage of a written exam.

The NCTRC also offers specialty certification in five areas of practice:

Behavioral health recreational therapy

Geriatric recreational therapy

Physical medicine and rehabilitation

Developmental disabilities recreational therapy

Community inclusion services

These specialty certifications can be earned through a combination of extensive experience in the field, continuing education credits, professional references, and graduate-level study in the area of specialization.

EARNINGS

THE AVERAGE YEARLY INCOME OF A RECREATIONAL therapist is about $50,000. That works out to almost $25 an hour. Those who are new to the field earn the least, with salaries ranging between $30,000 and $35,000. More experienced practitioners earn more than $60,000 a year, and those at the top of their field can earn more than $75,000. Actual earnings for any recreational therapist are determined by several factors: type of employer, geography, education level, and experience.

Employment Setting

The place of work is the single most important factor in determining a recreational therapist's salary. As with most jobs, the bigger the employer the bigger the paycheck. The government is the biggest employer of all. On average, recreational therapists who work for the government earn $57,000 a year. However, not all government facilities pay this well. The Veterans Affairs Administration, for example, offers an average of $49,000.

Hospitals represent the second largest employer of recreational therapists. This includes facilities that provide general medical services, surgery, and psychiatric care. Overall, recreational therapists who work in hospitals earn an average of $50,000. The size of the facility and of its parent company can make a big difference. A large urban hospital owned by one of the big national corporations is going to be able to offer more money than a small community hospital in a rural area.

Of the major employers, assisted living and skilled nursing care facilities for the elderly pay the lowest wages. Unlike large hospitals that have many patients generating revenue, these facilities are generally small with few paying patients. Those who work in these settings earn about $40,000 a year, which is less than the average for all recreational therapists.

Geographic Location

The rule of thumb is: the bigger the population, the bigger the paycheck. A recreational therapist in a big city is going to earn more than one in a rural area because the more residents there are, the more demand there is for services.

Recreational therapist salaries also vary by region. The highest wages are offered on the West Coast and in the Northeast. At the top of the list is California, with an average yearly salary of $65,000. Salaries are also especially good in Connecticut, New York, and New Jersey. The average earnings in these states are around $56,000 annually. Because of the high concentration of government facilities in the District of Columbia, salaries are a little higher there. Arizona is also a good location for recreational therapists. This is mostly because of the large number of retirees. The lowest wages are found in the Central Plains states and the South. It should be noted that the cost of living tends to level the field.

Education

It is possible to enter the career with a two-year associate degree but this is the minimum education level and salaries reflect that. Recreational therapists with a four-year bachelor's degree earn considerably more, and they have the added advantage of being eligible for promotions. A recreational therapist with an associate degree is stuck in a low-paying position until more education is obtained.

Salaries are even higher for those with advanced degrees. A master's degree or doctorate opens the door to supervisory roles and the opportunity to work in research.

Experience

Salaries also rise with experience. An experienced professional with 20 years in the field can earn three times the salary of a new graduate with less than a year on the job.

OPPORTUNITIES

THE FUTURE LOOKS BRIGHT FOR JOB seeking recreational therapists. Job growth has been accelerating over the past few years, and government experts now predict a 12 percent growth rate over the coming decade. That is faster than the average for all occupations.

The primary reason for the growing demand is the aging population. The US population has been aging steadily ever since the first Baby Boomer hit retirement age. Older people are naturally more subject to injuries and illnesses. Recreational therapists can help treat people who suffer from strokes, Alzheimer's disease, and mobility-related and age-related illnesses and injuries. The growing need for services will create more jobs in nursing care facilities, adult daycare programs, and other settings for geriatric patients. These employers already account for a third of all job opportunities. Recreational therapists who specialize in working with the elderly, and especially those who are certified in geriatric therapy, will have the best job prospects.

Baby Boomers are known for their desire to remain active, both socially and physically. There are a number of ways that recreational therapists can help seniors improve their health and maintain their independence. For example, older people are more at risk for falls than the general population. Falls for these people can be much more serious than a bump and bruise, especially when osteoporosis is present (an age-related condition). In fact, hip fractures can lead to premature death. Recreational therapists can help prevent falls by teaching modified yoga exercises that improve balance and strength. The same instruction can also slow the progression of osteoporosis. Because hospitals stays are getting shorter and people prefer to age at home, there will be more job opportunities in outpatient and community-based settings.

Recreational therapists can also help people with chronic conditions. This is a growing area of healthcare. Nearly half the entire population is afflicted by diabetes, obesity, chronic pain, and other long-term disabilities. Recreational therapists can help patients maintain their mobility, manage their conditions, and engage in healthy recreational activities that are adjusted to meet any physical limitations. They are uniquely qualified to plan and lead programs designed to improve mental and physical health through activities such as sports, dance, swimming, and camps. Many of the new job openings will arise from state-sponsored programs and local community centers. Schools may be hiring more recreational therapists as well, due to new laws requiring services for students with disabilities.

The VA will continue to be a major employer of recreational therapists. More and more recreational therapists are needed to help veterans manage service-related conditions like post-traumatic stress disorder (PTSD) and life-changing injuries such as the loss of a limb. Recreational therapy can help veterans reenter their communities and adjust to any physical, social, or cognitive limitations.

Despite the positive outlook, there will be competition for the best jobs. Although you can enter the field with a two-year associate degree, job prospects will be much greater for recreational therapists who earn a bachelor's degree in therapeutic recreation. For an additional advantage, getting credentialed as a Certified Therapeutic Recreation Specialist (CTRS) is highly recommended. Also highly valued are specialized certifications such as aquatic therapy, meditation, or crisis intervention. Look at where the need is greatest. For example, recreational therapists are still widely used in medical facilities such as spinal rehabilitation hospitals where quadriplegics need complicated activities.

Recreational therapists might experience more competition for jobs in certain regions of the country. Demand is generally greater in highly populated areas, so recreational therapists who are willing to relocate may have the best job prospects.

Recreational therapy aides are also in great demand, particularly in nursing homes and elementary schools where complicated therapeutic techniques are not usually needed. Aides do not have a degree, are typically just out of high school, and earn minimum wage. It is a good place to start and get a real feel for what the work is all about, but without the education that recreational therapists have, there is no path to advancement.

GETTING STARTED

ASIDE FROM A GOOD EDUCATION, what employers of recreational therapists like to see most is experience. You can start getting that experience while still in school. One of the best ways is through internships. Internship programs are very common among hospitals. They are also widely available through rehabilitation centers of all kinds, nursing homes, and some types of community health centers. You can find internship opportunities posted in your school's career placement center, or you can simply ask your counselor for help finding them. Intern programs for undergraduates typically last about 10 weeks and are usually scheduled during the summer months. Some offer compensation, some do not. Regardless, the experience is extremely valuable to your future goals.

There can be competition getting into an internship. Most students understand the value of these programs and many schools require participation in at least one internship to graduate. While you are working on getting into an internship, make good use of your time doing volunteer work. It looks just as good on a résumé as interning and is actually the most common way new recreational therapists gain experience. One big advantage to volunteer work is that it can be found anywhere, even in your hometown when you are home during summer breaks. To find volunteer opportunities, look in the same type of places where you would expect to find internships.

Continue to look for internships after graduation. The goal at this point is a little different. You will still be getting valuable experience, but you are also looking to land your first job. Employers routinely offer internships to new graduates to try them out. If it is a good fit, it can lead to a permanent job offer. Post-graduate internships can be offered at any time (not just during summer break) and may last for a few months up to a couple of years.

Stake out your area of specialization. Employers often look for candidates with experience in their field of practice, such as pediatrics, mental health, or rehabilitation. If you are looking for work in a big city, you will probably be able to pick and choose a specialty that interests you most. If not, you might have to work as a generalist, for a while at least. Plan ahead. Focus your attention on internships, volunteer work, and training in your chosen specialty.

Start networking early. Your list of contacts should include college professors and supervisors from intern or volunteer work. Join professional organizations and actively participate to get your name out there. Add your best contacts to your list of references on your résumé.

There are several good places to look for jobs. Start at your school's career center. Listings are posted regularly along with notices of any upcoming job fairs. Professional associations just for recreational therapists usually post jobs on their websites. Start with the American Therapeutic Recreation Association (ATRA), which maintains a job database devoted to recreational therapist jobs. Do not overlook all the associations devoted to specialty areas. There are also employment agencies, both on the Internet and off, that specialize in healthcare related jobs.

You can also look for unadvertised job openings. Go straight to the source and apply directly to hospitals, rehabilitation centers, nursing homes, school districts, and anywhere else that hires recreational therapists. There may not be any openings at the time you apply, but your résumé will be kept on file and reviewed when one comes up.

ASSOCIATIONS

■ **American Therapeutic Recreation Association**
https://www.atra-online.com

■ **National Council for Therapeutic Recreation Certification**
http://nctrc.org

■ **American Music Therapy Association**
https://www.musictherapy.org

■ **American Art Therapy Association**
https://arttherapy.org

■ **American Dance Therapy Association**
https://adta.org

PERIODICALS

■ **The Therapeutic Recreation Journal**
https://js.sagamorepub.com/trj

■ **American Journal of Recreation Therapy**
http://www.pnpco.com

WEBSITES

■ **Recreational Therapy – Mayo Clinic School of Health Services**
http://www.mayo.edu/mayo-clinic
-school-of-health-sciences/careers
/recreational-therapy

■ **RecreationTherapy.com**
https://www.recreationtherapy.com

www.ingramcontent.com/pod-product-compliance
Lightning Source LLC
Chambersburg PA
CBHW070521220526
45467CB00002B/783